I0845104

Best book for HEALTHY
Lifestle & Emergency
Medicine

WHAT YOUR BODY TELLS ABOUT YOU.

food facts and managent of

chronic diseases

EMERGENCY CASES IN INTERNAL MEDICINE.

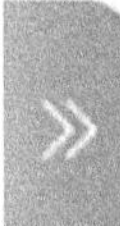

COLLINS N.C MD
PHYSICIAN

FORWARD

Because the landscape of medication maintains to adapt, this textbook will serve as a steadfast partner, guiding you through the challenges and triumphs that lie in advance in your adventure as a healthcare expert. Whether you're a pupil embarking on your educational odyssey or a skilled clinician seeking to live at the leading edge of scientific understanding, this textbook is designed to support you in your pursuit of excellence.

I extend my heartfelt appreciation to the authors, editors, and everybody worried inside the advent of this useful aid. Their commitment to improving medical training and affected person care shines brightly through the pages of this textbook.

may additionally this textbook ignite your passion for internal medicinal drugs and inspire you to make a profound distinction within the lives of those you serve. together, allow us to embrace the artwork and technological know-how of medication with compassion, humility, and unwavering determination. Also there lots of information about dieting and chronic disease

DEDICATION

THIS BOOK is dedicated to God almighty the maker of heaven and earth and my lovely parents who made all the sacrifices so i can graduate successfully from Medical university. I Dedicate this book to all medical students and those who aspire to be a health professional .

TABLE OF CONTENTS

EMERGENCY TREATMENT OF MI (MYOCARDIUM INFARCTION)

Myocardial infarction (MI), WHICH IS KNOWN AS "heart attack," is caused by REDUCTION or complete cessation of blood flow to a portion of the myocardium. Myocardial infarction may be"silent," and go undetected, or it could be a calamitous event leading to hemodynamic deterioration and sudden death.

TREAMENT

Supplementary oxygen (if Sao2 less than 90%.
* aspirin 325 mg
* Clopidogrel inhibits platelets aggregation 600 mg plus daily 75 mg
* sublingual nitrates 0.4 mg neutral glycerin ABSORPTION IS RAPID
 causes RELAXATION of smooth muscles dilation of vessels
 *Beta blockers: (if hypotension, bradycardia do not give and COPD
*High dose of starting 80 mg
 anticoagulation Heparin 300 ml single those- 1000-2500IU

If symptoms Persist Give IV: nitroglycerin 7.5-30 mg
IV morphine for severe pain: 2.5-15 mg
Unstable sinus bradycardia and low blood pressure IV
atropine 2 mg which blocks parasympathetic nervous
system

 if pulmonary edema IV Furosemide 20-80 mg

REPERFUSION

1 CORONARY ANGIOPLASTY , Place a balloon or mesh
on blocked artery if this is not available
 thrombolysis **streptokinase** to break this stenosis and
make way for a bypass surgery
To avoid stents thrombosis fatal complication of stenting;
dual antiplatelet therapy must be used (Aspirin and
Clopidogrel.

EMERGENCY TREATMENT FOR CARDIOGENIC SHOCK
*Intense fatigue, cold sweaty, Confucian, chest pain, Rapids weak
Heartbeats, Fainting, oligonuria,* Causes: *fluid around hearts,
pulmonary embolism, c a d, valve damage, Hearts muscles
arrhythmia.*

Blood test ECG, echocardiogram, cardiac catheterization, if
blocked or narrow artery oxygen supplementation, If
arrhythmia use defibrillator to convert the heart rhythm of
the heart,
 restore blood pressure dopamine, epinephrine 20 to 50
Mcg/ kg mm

aspirin + Clopidogrel immediately
then continue from the Mi treatment pattern.

Extracorporeal membrane oxygenation:Helps improve
blood flow and supplies oxygen to the body, blood is
pumped outside of your body to a heart lungs machine that
removes carbon dioxide and sends oxygen filled blood
back to the tissue in the body.
Heart injury repair. Heart assist devices and transplant.

ELECTRICAL DEFIBRILLATOR: IS A device that sends
an electric pulse or signal to the hearts to restore or
prevent an arrhythmia. For slow or fast Heart Beat even if
the heart has stopped this will help it beat again .Wearable
cardioverter defibrillator and implantable cardioverter
defibrillator ICD.

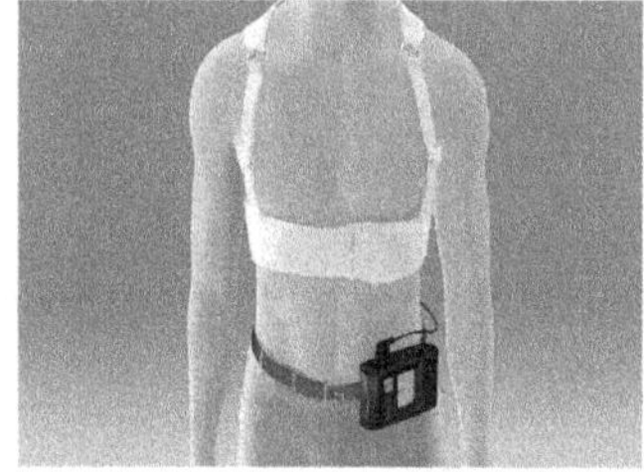

wearable cardioverter defibrillator.

HOW IT WORKS:An electric current goes from
negative to positive electrode of defibrillator and passes
to the hearts, this induces transmembrane potential in
myocardial cells and results in synchronizing the
polarization of all myocardium.

STERNAL PUNCTURE BIOPSY, TECHNIQUE, INDICATION AND CONTRAINDICATION.

INDICATIONS: Anemia, cancer, fevers of Unknown Origin, hemochromatosis.

PROCEDURE:

LOCAL Anastasia, clean the area with antiseptics,Inserts a Hulu needle through the bone into the bone marrow and using the syringe take out bone marrow,

usually done in 2-3 ICS in mediastinum.

CONTRAINDICATION: Hemorrhagic fever (hemophilia d i c) long term use of anticoagulant, skin infection radiation therapy bone diseases osteomyelitis.

INTERPRETATION OF COAGULATION IN CARDIOLOGY

*Full blood counts   to look at platelets thrombocytopenia in case of platelet defects

* bleeding time———-------   measure platelet and Vascular response.

 *Prothrombin time   access extrinsic pathway of coagulation

 *activated partial thromboplastin time
Intrinsic pathway of coagulation

thrombin time   Fibrinogen to fibrin conversion

lipids   level of cholesterol .

ACUTE RENAL FAILURE /UREMIC COMA
Treats on the underlying cause
* correct blood volume
* Antibiotics

 Hyperkalemia: exogenous source is stopped
* dopamine Ca gluconate
,glucose

*if hypomagnesemia, give mg sulfate
 if severe acidosis—------give Na by carbonate
 *control BP and diuretics

***Dialysis: hemodialysis and peritoneal dialysis
INDICATION: if blood creatinine >0.7mm/l and CFR <
10m/mm/1.73
ANAPHYLACTIC SHOCK
Check ABC   give CPR if needed
 high flow oxygen
 Venous access
 Adrenaline 0.5 ml
 IV antihistamine and cortisol to decrease
inflammation and improve passage of air,
 B Agonist Albuterol to relieve breathing symptoms-
2.5 mg by nebulization

monitor vital signs, monitor water intake and urine output

for angioedema give Antihistamine oral steroid diphenhydramine and cetirizine

EMERGENCY TREATMENT FOR CARDIAC ASTHMA \PULMONARY EDEMA.

COMPLICATION OF CARDIAC FAILURE(FLUID BUILDUP)

Indication of congestive heart failure, (Arrhythmia , BP, diabetes , hyperthyroidism can cause cardiac asthma.

SIGNS AND SYMPTOMS

Trouble breathing, WHEEZING, coughing bloody or fruits sputum, rales, chest pain fatigue Blue color of skin, swelling in chest and Ankle fluid retention

ECG and Eco. and blood test.

TREATMENT: morphine10-25mg, nitroglycerine 0.4 mg or diuretics then surgery

IV furosemide nitroglycerine and morphine are used for acute treatment of cardiac asthma, if hypoxic supplementary oxygen.

EMERGENCY TREATMENT OF HYPERTENSIVE CRISIS.

A hypertensive crisis is a sudden, severe increase in blood pressure. The blood pressure reading is 180/120 millimeters of mercury (mm Hg) or greater. A hypertensive

crisis is a medical emergency. It can lead to a heart attack,
stroke or other life-threatening health problems
IS DIVIDED INTO TWO
- EMERGENCY, which lead to organ damage and
- URGENCY, without organ damage

Urgency treatment:
New organ damage
 Captopril 25 mg Max 50 mg
 clonidine 0.1- 0.2 mg Max those 0.8 mg
 0.1 every hour until achieve results
labetalol: 200 mg PO followed by 200 every hour marks
1,200 mg

Emergency treatment:
Nitroprusside if angina- Nitroglycerine 0.4 mg(sl)
Nicardipine-(20-40 mg)
If fluid retention, give IV furosemide/
Clevidipine (1-2 mg IV, max 32mg.)

Also diet is essential in the treatment of hypertension,
avoid salty diet and eat more plant base food , fruits and
vegetables and lots of fiber and iron rich food. Exercise and
avoid refined floor and white bread and meat.

HYPOTONIC AND VEGETATIVE -VASCULAR CRISES
If you have acute or severe hyponatremia it's emergency
options are
 Intravenous fluid; IV Sodium solution to slowly raise the
Na+ level in your blood, You are required to stay in the

hospital, Rapid of Correction is dangerous.(little administration)
MEDICATION: medication to manage signs and symptoms of hyponatremia such as Headache nausea and seizure.

EMERGENCY PAROXYSMAL TACHYCARDIA, ATRIAL FLUTTER.
 AND FIBRILLATION .
Most people terminate acute episodes of paroxysmal tachycardia by Vega Maneuvers, carotid massage.
 intravenous adenosine 12 mg those iv, is a safe efficacious treatment for the emergent treatment of tachycardia, also verapamil together calcium channel blockers VERAPIMIL 80-120 mg, 2-3 times a day…..

ATRIAL FLUTTER:
Treatment of acute arterial Florida width ivy dutyism 0.25 mg/ kg- 0.35 mg/ kg, ventricular heart rate WILL significantly decrease
Some cases,combine diltiazem+digoxin (8-12 mcg/kg

HEPATIC COMA
INTRAVENOUS Hydration and correction of any hypoglycemia or electrolyte disturbance.
Blood Ammonia lowering therapy : lactulose which helps reduce ammonia levels in the blood and also decrease intestinal production and absorption of ammonia , it draws ammonia from blood into the colon, where the body excrete it …LACTULOSE, LACTITOL.

BLEEDING FROM G.I.T

Upper GIT bleeding= melena -dark stool
Hematemesis- vomiting of bright red blood
Lower GIT-bringt red in stool.

GIT bleed: ulcers, H pylori, diverticular, IBD, hemorrhoid.
MEDICATION: NSAID, Anticoagulant, (aspirin+clopidogrel)
Check for renal disease and cancer.

Emergency: Airway= oxygen
Breathing -oxygen
Check for shock and signs of it, pulse IV-fluid crystalline, if anemic give blood.
CHECK blood count and liver functional test, after stabilization. Follow endoscopy
*heater probe , clip, adrenaline—-into the bleeding area, hemospray.

EMERGENCY TREATMENT OF PROFUSE DIARRHEA.

Stabilization of Passion by giving fluid and electrolytes imbalance treatment and quickly do test to deter the underlying cause: IV antimicrobial therapy. zinc and probiotics reduce severity.

BILIARY COLIC

Relief of symptoms and correction of any underlying cause, biliary Colic is abdominal pain due to obstruction usually by Stone in the cystic duct or common by ducts.

 Remove the pain

 opiate analgesics;meperidine 10 milligram/ ml

 Antiemetics- stop vomiting; promethazine- 25 mg.

Antispasmodic agent: glycopyrrolate

Then followed by surgery to remove the obstruction.

ACUTE PANCREATITIS

Most of the cases of pancreatitis in the emergency department are treated conservatively which is fluid resuscitation, pain management. morphine 0.1 mg/ IV, MEPERIDINE 10 mg/ IV

 sepsis control- use of antibiotics Ciprofloxacin 400 mg

EMERGENCY CARDIAC TAMPONADE ,PERICARDIOCENTESIS

Cardiac tamponade is often MEDICAL emergency and quick removal of the pericardial fluid is the most common procedure to do is called a pericardiocentesis; and you do it using long thin tube (A catheter Is used to remove the fluid using antibiotics and pain medication.

ASTHMA ATTACK/ ASTHMA STATUS

You have to bring the Asthma under control.
1, short acting beta agonist " Albuterol
2: intravenous corticosteroid : 40-60 mg better than Po
3:Ipratropium: is used as bronchodilator to treat a severe asthma attack
4: intubation, Mechanical ventilation and oxygen
Patient is watched for few hours and allowed to go home

SPONTANEOUS PNEUMOTHORAX TREATMENT

Is bed rest, oxygen therapy, observation, simple aspiration, close intercostal tube drainage and Tube thoracostomy.
 for tension pneumothorax needle is used for decompression, insert a long (14- 16) gauge needle into the second intercostal space in the midclavicular line -Air will usually go out

PULMONARY EMBOLISM

First oxygen therapy
 painkillers IV and flu therapy
 0.1 mg /kg morphine
 Heparin IV - 5,000 IU/ml max
1000-2000 units/hour
Warfarin orally=150 mg po
Thrombolytics=0.25mg-0. 9 mg/kg
Streptokinase- eminas
Nitroglycerine

CAUSES: Pneumothorax, pulmonary embolism,
right-heart failure, hemothorax, acute exacerbation
of diseases.
e, activase.

RESPIRATORY FAILURE EMERGENCY
TREATMENT
First is admitted to ICU; can be treated at home
with supplementary oxygen/ ventilator assist
devices- treatment of underlying diseases
 Airway management
 chest decompression
 bronchodilators/ steroid
 Epinephrine 0.5-1.0 mg
                    PULMONARY EDEMA
Oxygen therapy
 Sit patients with legs down
Nitroglycerin sublingually

+morphine

Furosemide IV, decrease blood volume-

EMERGENCY TREATMENT FOR BLAST CRISIS.

A life threatening hematologic emergency, increase in blood cells in Marrow result in blood hyperviscosity and relatively reduction of other cells, decrease in tissue Perfusion via forming white cells plugs in microvasculature

Symptoms; weakness, fatigue, night sweats, weight loss, fever, bone pain, abdominal fullness.

Tissue Perfusion: —decrease blood flow, stroke like symptoms

Management: aggressive treatment of any sign of infection with broad spectrum antibiotics.

Anemia should be treated with packed Rbc and diuretics can worsen the viscosity of blood.

LEUKOSTASIS: WHICH IS ALSO an emergency situation, LEUKAPHERESIS IS INDICATED..

HEMORRHAGIC DIATHESIS

Hemophilia types

Bleeding diathesis presents;— easy bruises, gum bleeding, nosebleeds, Petaches, purpura, excessive bleeding after small cuts, tooth extraction, blood in urine, stool, vomiting

blood transfusion;- fresh frozen plasma, packed RBC
synthetic clothing Factor.

HEMORRHAGIC SHOCK: HYPOVOLEMIC
ABC- Stop bleeding
High flow oxygen.
=venous access
Monitor vital signs= pulse, Bp, Spo2, RR
Monitor ECG
Linen cather
IV crystalloid , blood transfusion .
Drugs to increase pump: dopamin, epinephrine, dobutamine , norepinephrine.

HEMOLYTIC CRISIS
When large amount of red blood cell is destroyed, CAUSING
jaundice , liver and spleen enlargement, fever

Detoxification methods
Hemo-transfusion in severe degree
steroids

Autoimmune infection can lead to hemolytic crisis .
 treat the underlying disease cause, blood
transfusion and corticosteroid therapy .

END OF THE EMERGENCY CASES.
WHAT YOUR BODY TELLS ABOUT YOUR
HEALTH

1: DARK CIRCLE AROUND YOUR EYES; It shows
you have a problem with insulin resistance.

2;If you're getting big bags under your eyes, that's a
little bit of swelling under your eyes that is related to
sluggish kidney or poor kidney function.

3: but if you have Bloody eyes, it's related to
insufficiency of the liver or Poor Liver Health
4: if you're getting cracks in the corner of your mouth
it shows lack of vitamins especially vitamin C and
due to deficiency of vitamin B6
5: if you're getting a lot of black hair on your face is
a result of vitamin D deficiency
6 if you have a lot of acne is a result of poor gut
health or food sensitivity.
    ABOUT THE TONGUE
A pink tongue is healthy and normal. A red tongue
may indicate heat in the body like a fever or a
hormonal imbalance. A reddish purple tongue is a

sign that there may be inflammation or an infection in the body. A pale pink tongue may be a sign of a vitamin deficiency, a weak immune system or a lack of energy.

ABOUT THE NAIL.
A touch of white here, a rosy tinge there, or some rippling or bumps may be a sign of disease in the body. Problems in the liver, lungs, and heart can show up in your nails

ABOUT POOP, (FECES)

1: BLOODY STOOL(feces) dark , sign of laceration, tear, perforation or ulcer of upper digestive system,
Fresh red, sign of polyps, tear of lower digestive tract, report to Doctor or call emergency.

2:HARD STOOL(FECES): sign of constipation, low fiber or excessive consumption of baked floor, and carbs. Can cause tear of the anus .

3: WATERY STOOL: DEPEND ON THE TYPE AND SEVERITY : is a sign of diarrhea , if it is bloody, call emergency immediately ; and if (rice water sign of .CHOLERA. If you visit the toilet more than thrice, more than two days, seek medical help.

BASIC HERBAL REMEDY FOR GOOD HEALTH AND LONGEVITY.

If you don't eat your food like medicine, you will end up eating medicine like food.

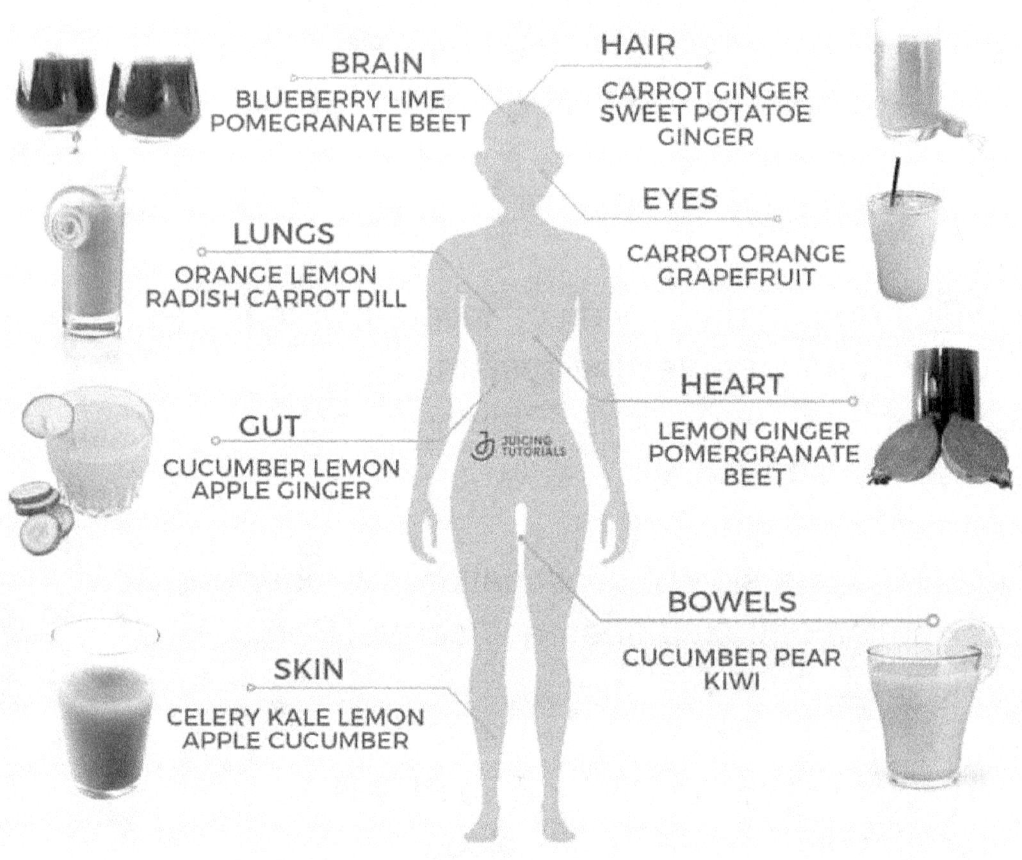

IF WANT TO LOSE WEIGHT AND BE FIT, EAT WHEN THE SUN RISE AND STOP EATING AFTER THE SUN GOES DOWN. 11AM-6PM

Zobo leaf,Cinnamon lemon and ginger smash it, Pineapple peal, lemongrass gloves, pineapple and add little honey to it.

FOOD FACTS THAT YOU HAVE TO KNOW

Taking a hot Ginger drink after your meal makes you Fuller for a long period of time. is a great remedy for weight loss

2* Orange fruits like carrots sweet potato orange itself tangerine are good for the eyesight

3* eating two kiwi before bedtime helps you sleep faster and better

4* Pineapple juice is stronger in stopping cough and stopping cough that cough syrup itself

5 Taking cashew nuts with honey increases brain memory,

6 eating for strawberries daily lowest bad cholesterol improves vision and prevent heart attack

7 sweet potato contains lots of vitamin A; it gives a healthy skin and impulse eye function

8; Eating cucumbers before bedtime improves sleep. It helps you wake up refreshed and headache free.

9; Two bananas will give you enough energy for
2 hours of workouts

10 ; apples are more effective in waking you up
than a cup of coffee

FOODS THAT SHOULD BE EATEN TOGETHER

APPLE + DARK CHOCOLATE

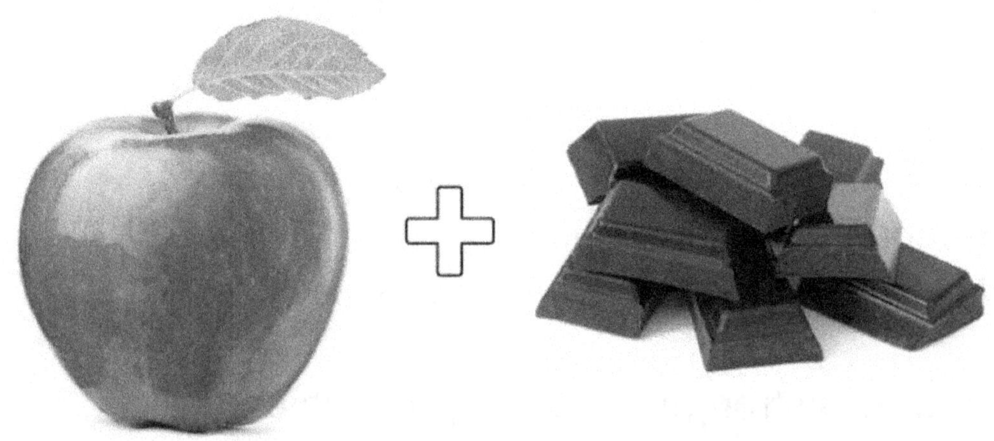

AN ANTI-INFLAMMATORY CRUCIAL TO HEART HEALTH
FOUND IN APPLES AND POWERFUL ANTIOXIDANTS FOUND IN
DARK CHOCOLATE FORMS A TASTY SNACK THAT FIGHTS
BLOOD COTS, IMPROVES CIRCULATION AND REDUCES YOUR
CHANCES OF HEART DISEASE.

LEMON + KALE

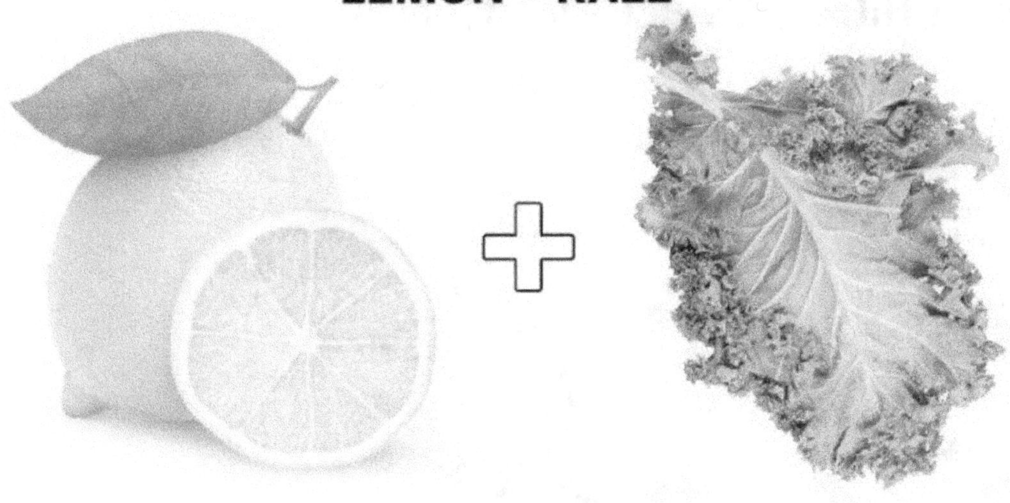

VITAMIN C (HIGHLY ABUNDANT IN LEMONS) MAKES PLANT-BASED IRON(SUCH AS IRON-RICH KALE) MORE ABSORBABLE IN THE BODY

LEMON + GREEN TEA

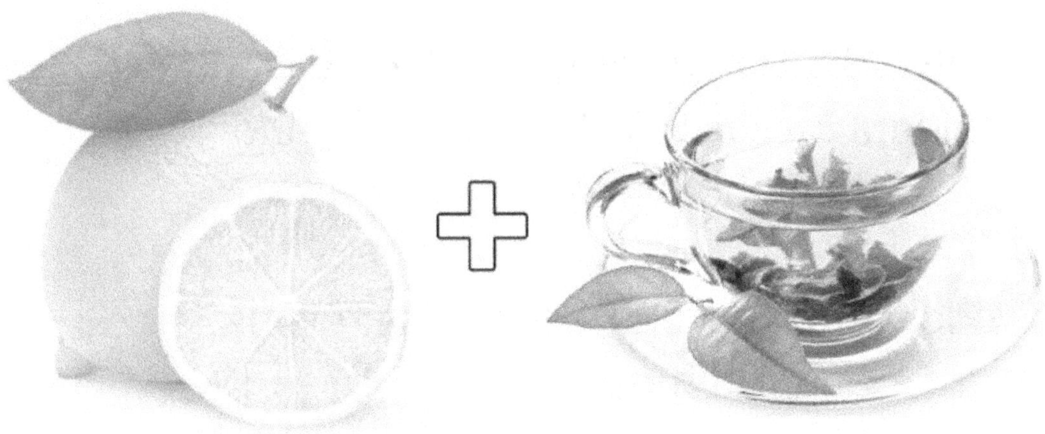

ADDING LEMON TO A CUP OF GREEN TEA ALLOWS THE BODY TO ABSORB THE ANTIOXIDANTS FROM THE GREEN TEA MORE EFFECTIVELY. THESE ARE KNOWN AS CATECHINS AND THEY ARE RESPONSIBLE FOR MOST HEALTH BENEFITS OF GREEN TEA.

CHICKPEA + BEET ROOT

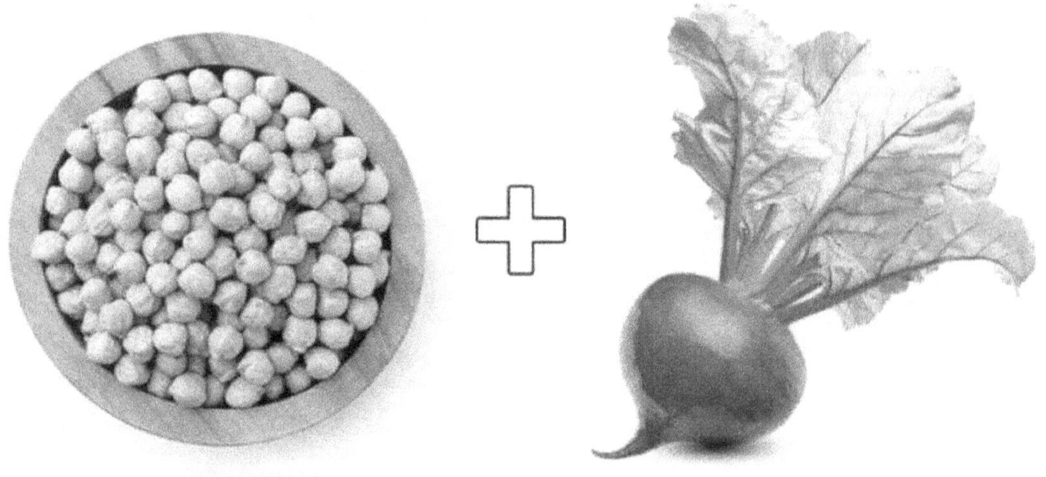

CHICKPEAS ARE RICH IN VITAMIN B6, A VITAMIN THAT HELPS THE BODY ABSORB MAGNESIUM-RICH FOODS LIKE BEETS.

MORE THINGS TO KNOW ABOUT FOOD

If you cant sleep MAGNESIUM; avocado and dark chocolate

IF you have low energy you need IRON;raisins and red meat.

IF you feel weak you need zinc:MANGO

IF you wake up tired you need potassium:coconut water.

HOW TO MAKE WINE AT HOME:

PINEAPPLE, CINAMON, AND HIBISCUS FLOWER, BOIL FOR TEN MINUTES AND ENJOY.

HOME REMEDY FOR HIGH BLOOD PRESSURE

Coconut water and mix with lime, remedy and it will help lower your BP.

HOW TO GET A GLOWING SKIN/ MAKE YOUR SKIN LOOK BETTER AND YOUNGER

INGREDIENTS : 1

1* ALOE VERA

2* BANANA

3* HONEY

4*AVOCADO

5: WHITE PART OF EGG(BOILED EGG)

So you have to blend all together and remember the egg must be boiled, put the white part, .

Put it in a container and store it in the refrigerator . three times a day, rub after shower at night and in the morning, rinse your body with warm water, NOTE You have to skip a day after each application, meaning: if you apply on monday, next will be wednesday, next friday, after two weeks you stop.

REFERENCES:
1: all materials mostly from gomel state medical university.
2: mayoclinic
4: clevelandclinic.org
5:medscape.com
6: my personal knowledge i have gathered all my life as a medical professional